Laetitia MONDAKO MAKOMBI

Level of knowledge about tuberculosis among the population

Laetitia MONDAKO MAKOMBI

Level of knowledge about tuberculosis among the population

IN KINSHASA 2019

ScienciaScripts

Imprint
Any brand names and product names mentioned in this book are subject to trademark, brand or patent protection and are trademarks or registered trademarks of their respective holders. The use of brand names, product names, common names, trade names, product descriptions etc. even without a particular marking in this work is in no way to be construed to mean that such names may be regarded as unrestricted in respect of trademark and brand protection legislation and could thus be used by anyone.

Cover image: www.ingimage.com

This book is a translation from the original published under ISBN 978-620-6-73496-3.

Publisher:
Sciencia Scripts
is a trademark of
Dodo Books Indian Ocean Ltd. and OmniScriptum S.R.L publishing group

120 High Road, East Finchley, London, N2 9ED, United Kingdom
Str. Armeneasca 28/1, office 1, Chisinau MD-2012, Republic of Moldova, Europe
Managing Directors: Ieva Konstantinova, Victoria Ursu
info@omniscriptum.com

Printed at: see last page
ISBN: 978-620-6-17208-6

SUMMARY

Context

Tuberculosis is a veritable scourge throughout the world. Public awareness of this disease is a key factor in reducing contamination and the associated death rate.

Objective

The aim of this study was to contribute to improving the management of tuberculosis in the provincial city of Kinshasa by assessing the population's level of knowledge about this disease.

Methods

Cross-sectional, descriptive study involving 300 randomly selected respondents from 4 churches in the city of Kinshasa. Sociodemographic characteristics and knowledge of tuberculosis were studied.

Results

Of the 300 people surveyed, 53.3% were women with an average age of 30.4±11.9 years. Among them, 45.3% had a low socio-economic status. One hundred percent of respondents were informed about tuberculosis; the medical profession and the media were the main sources of information. Overall good knowledge of tuberculosis was 15%. Knowledge was significantly higher among civil servants (p=0.048), Protestants and Kimbanguists (p=0.007).

Conclusion

Overall knowledge of tuberculosis is low in the study population, despite the information received from the medical profession and the media about the disease. Raising awareness through other channels, such as the community, could improve this knowledge.

Keywords: Knowledge, tuberculosis, Kinshasa

TABLE OF CONTENTS

SUMMARY 1

EPIGRAPH 4

DEDICATION 5

ACKNOWLEDGEMENTS 6

ABBREVIATIONS 7

INTRODUCTION 9

CHAPTER 1. GENERAL INFORMATION 13

CHAPTER 2. MATERIALS AND METHODS 29

CHAPTER 3. RESULTS 32

CHAPTER 4. DISCUSSION 40

CONCLUSION 43

RECOMMENDATIONS 44

REFERENCES 46

APPENDIX 50

EPIGRAPH

"Again I have seen under the sun that the race is not to the nimble, nor war to the valiant, nor bread to the wise, nor riches to the clever, nor favor to the learned; for all depends for them on time and circumstances." Ecclesiastes 9:11d

DEDICATION

I affectionately dedicate this work to my husband MPONA-MINGA SHAMBA, the father of my beloved son; to my father Raphael MAKOMBI, to my mother Rose MPEMBE and to my beloved older brother Charly MBEMBE-YONGO MAKOMBI.

They believed in me from my very first steps in medical school, they supported and encouraged me, and above all they showered me with love without ever tiring of it, despite the many difficulties.

To my brothers Fils MAKOMBI, Junior MAKOMBI, Franchou MAKOMBI, Guy MAKOMBI, Viana MAKOMBI, Emmanuel MAKOMBI, Guyguy MPIA, Guy BODO, Papy MPEMBE and sisters Séraphine MPIA, Nelly NKOTO, Judith GIMARANZI and Judith LIBANA.

ACKNOWLEDGEMENTS

On the threshold of this work, which marks the end of my studies in general medicine, I would like to express my deep gratitude:

- To Almighty God, author of all grace, without whom this work would not be possible;
- To Professor Dr. AKETI Loukia, for directing this work, giving of himself for us in spite of his multiple occupations, and this with great dedication;
- To the authorities of the Faculty of Medicine at the University of Kinshasa;
- To Dr. Aliocha NKODILA for his availability for statistical analysis improvement of this work.
- To Professors; supervisors and assistants in Unit D of the Department of Pediatrics;
- To my very dear and loving husband MPONA-MINGA SHAMBA Nathanaël, may the Almighty remember you and bless you for your great love, your great heart, your great patience and your great support.
- To my brothers: Charly MAKOMBI, Fils MAKOMBI, Junior MAKOMBI, Franchou MAKOMBI, Guy MAKOMBI, Viana MAKOMBI, Emmanuel MAKOMBI, Guyguy MPIA, Guy BODO, Papy MPEMBE and sisters Séraphine MPIA, Nelly NKOTO, Judith GIMARANZI and Judith LIBANA.
- To my cousins, nephews and nieces: thank you for believing in me.
- To my in-laws: Dad, Mom and all the MPONA-MINGA family: thank you for your presence, your support and your love for me.
- We can't end this stage without mentioning a certain category of special people for what they are in my life: Mr and Mrs PATAULI, Audrey MUNDINE and all the MUNDINEs, Belinda MOYA and all the MOYAs, Grace LOMBO, Lord LOMBO, Nathalie NKOY, Marthe DELO, Pamela NGANA.
- Many thanks to my fellow fighters: Merveille KANKONDE, Laurinda MVUMBI, Zelda KINKELA, Naomie ALIMA, Souzy NGWEY, Thoria MONSHENIE, Dieudonné MWANGALA, Hornelly LUSAVUVU and all the others I couldn't name. You have made a great contribution to my life, and particularly to this work.
- To all those who have contributed in one way or another to my training, from elementary school to this level, please accept, with these few words, the expression of my gratitude.

ABBREVIATIONS

AB	Antibiotic
ANTI-T	Antituberculosis
Anti-TNF	Anti tumor necrosis factor
ARV	Antiretrovirals
BCG	Bacille Calmette et Guérin
BK	Koch's Bacile
CBCO	Communauté Baptiste au Congo
CBFC	Communauté Baptiste du Fleuve Congo
Coll	Associates
DS	Diabetes mellitus
Hab.	Inhabitant
IDR	Intradermal reaction
INH	Isoniazid
IR	Renal failure
ITL	Latent Tuberculosis Infection
MDR-TB	Multidrug-resistant tuberculosis
MICS	Multiple Indicator Cluster Survey
MT	Mycobacterium Tuberculosis
NC	New Case
NSE	Socioeconomic level
Nne	Newborn
WHO	World Health Organization
PCR	Polymerase Chain Reaction
Ph	Hydrogen potential

NMLS	Programme National Multisectoriel de Lutte contre le Sida
Pre-XDR	Pre-extensive multi-resistance
PHAS	Person living with HIV
GROUND	
FLOOR	Democratic Republic of Congo
Sd	Syndrome
Sero -	Negative
Sero +	HIV-positive
AIDS	Acquired immunodeficiency syndrome
TA	Active Tuberculosis
TB	Tuberculosis
TCT	Tuberculin skin test
TLIG	Interferon gamma release test
TPM	Tuberculosis Lung Disease
Tx.	Rates
USA	United State Of America
HIV	Human Immunodeficiency Virus
Vit B6	Vitamin B6
Vit K	Vitamin K
XDR	Extensive multi-resistance

INTRODUCTION

1. Context

Tuberculosis (TB) is a contagious, severe, often airborne, endemo-epidemic disease with essentially human-to-human transmission. It is caused by the *Mycobacterium tuberculosis* (MT) or bacillus Koch (BK) complex, which includes MT *hominis*, MT *bovis* and MT *africanum*. Pulmonary involvement is the most frequent localization, and represents the usual source of transmission. However, the bacillus can spread to other organs, resulting in extra-pulmonary TB. It is the second leading cause of death from infectious diseases worldwide, after infection with the human immunodeficiency virus (HIV/AIDS)(1).

The incidence of TB varies throughout the world, from low levels of between 0 and 9.9 per 100,000 inhabitants per year in Western countries (North America and Europe), to extremely high levels of over 500 per 100,000 inhabitants per year in South Africa. The continents most affected are Africa and South-East Asia (2).

Since 1986, TB has been on the increase worldwide. It was in the United States of America (USA) that the increase in the number of cases was reported (3% in 1986, 6% in 1990), and the role of HIV/AIDS infection in this resurgence appeared very likely. In Black Africa and South-East Asia, the extent of the tuberculosis endemic and the high prevalence of HIV/AIDS infection made this situation more frequent than elsewhere. As early as the first studies carried out in Central and East Africa, a rate (Tx) of TB-HIV co-infection equal to or greater than 30% was noted. Since 1994, a second serious factor has been added to HIV infection: resistance to anti-tuberculosis drugs (ANTI-T), resulting in multi-drug-resistant TB and extensively drug-resistant TB (3).

Lack of funds jeopardizes efforts to combat the global TB epidemic. Approximately US$2.3 billion of the US$9.2 billion investment required in 2017 in low- and middle-income countries is needed for care and prevention. In addition, at least another US$1.2 billion is needed each year to accelerate the development of new vaccines, diagnostics and drugs.

The World TB Report 2016 emphasizes two major challenges to making decisive progress in care and prevention, namely, drug-resistant TB and TB linked to HIV/AIDS infection. Multidrug-resistant TB continues to be a major public health crisis and a threat to health security. The World Health Organization (WHO) estimates that 600,000 new cases (NC) are rifampicin-resistant, of which 490,000 are multidrug-resistant. Three countries bear the main burden of this disease: India, China and Russia, accounting for almost half of all cases worldwide.

It is the leading cause of death among people living with HIV (PLHIV). TB-HIV co-infected subjects are 20 to 30 times more likely to develop progressive TB than HIV-negative(-) subjects. In 2016, there were 1.4 million TB NC in HIV-positive (sero +) individuals, 74% of whom lived in Africa. Forty percent of deaths among PLHIV are due to TB.

North Africa accounted for 20.5%, Central Africa for 12.9%, West Africa for 11.7%, East Africa for 8.2%, Southeast Asia for 15%, Eastern Europe for 12.7%, Southern Europe for 7.4%, Asia, Western Europe and North America for 1.5% of these TB cases in 2013 (2).

In the same year, WHO estimates that 9 million people contracted the disease and 1.5 million died, including 360,000 HIV-positive subjects (HIV+). The disease is slowly receding every year, and it is estimated that 37 million lives were saved between 2000 and 2013 thanks to effective treatment and diagnosis (1).

The 2016 Global TB Control Report reveals figures that remain as alarming as ever. In 2016, there were 10.4 million NCs worldwide (8.6 million in 2012 and 9.6 million in 2014). Six countries account for 64% of the total burden: India is the most affected, followed by Indonesia, China, the Philippines, Russia, Nigeria and South Africa. The 1.7 million people died in 2016 (1.3 million in 2012 and 1.5 million in 2014), including almost 400,000 co-infected with HIV. The increase in the number of NCs shows, in fact, an improvement in data collection. Over 53 million lives have been saved since 2000. But of the estimated 10.4 million TB sufferers, only 6.3 were diagnosed and officially notified in 2016, meaning that 4.1 million cases remained undiagnosed and therefore untreated, almost half of them in India, Indonesia and Nigeria. Globally, incidence is falling by around 2% a year. This rate must rise to reach 4% to 5% by 2020, to meet the first milestone of the WHO Strategy to End TB. The risk is higher in HIV+ subjects or those suffering from conditions that lead to reduced immunity (including smoking, which increases the risk of progressive TB: it is involved in 8% of TB cases worldwide) (1).

The WHO estimates that between 2000 and 2020, nearly a billion people will be newly infected with the TB bacillus, and that 200 million of them will develop TB, 35 million of whom will die if no progress is made in controlling the infection.

In children, the 2011 estimate was 500,000 cases, including 5.7% of cases in children under 15, and 64,000 deaths, including 6.5% of HIV+ children. In 2013, of the 9 million TB-related cases, 550,000 were children aged 0-15, 80,000 of whom were HIV+. In the same year, in the USA, 9,582 cases of TB were reported, of which 485 or 5% were children under 15 (3).

2. Justification

The Democratic Republic of Congo (DRC) is one of the 22 most TB-affected countries in the world, ranking 5th in Africa and 10th worldwide (4).

In the DRC, an estimated 36,000 TB-related deaths occur every year, 28% of which are attributable to HIV (5).

WHO estimated that, in 2003, the annual incidence of TB in the DRC was 160 cases per 100,000 population. Since 1987, this number has been rising steadily, from 15,000 cases of pulmonary TB disease (PDT) in 1987 to 62,519 in 2004. This increase is partly attributable to HIV infection, with an average prevalence of 4.3% (PNMLS, 2008).

Childhood TB accounts for approximately 15-40% of all TB cases and is usually acquired through contact with an infecting adult. High transmission rates are encountered in endemic areas due to high population density and long delays in diagnosis. In 2000, according to the WHO, 6.3 million people were diagnosed with TB, 10% of whom were children under the age of 15 (6).

Several factors have been identified as risk factors for the disease. In some studies, patients with recent contact (< 2 years) with TB (10%), illegal residents (8.5%), asylum seekers (7.8%), the homeless (3.7%) and prisoners (2.2%) have been identified as risk groups (7).

These factors have a variable influence on the risk of progression to TB. However, other factors were present in varying proportions: immunodepression in 5.6% of cases, chronic alcoholism in 5.5% of cases, HIV in 3.7% of cases, diabetes in 3.3% of cases, pulmonary fibrotic lesions in 2% of cases, renal failure (IR) in 1.9% of cases, pneumoconiosis in 1.3% of cases and intravenous drug abuse in 1% of cases (4). HIV and its immunosuppression is an important factor in the acquisition and progression of TB. In Holland, between 2002 and 2014, there were almost 25 cases per year of TB-HIV co-infection, 25 times more than the national average (22% Dutch and 78% non-Dutch) (3).

The discovery of TB must be followed by systematic HIV screening, which is not yet the case everywhere. In Belgium, in 2012, patients with TB associated or not with HIV averaged 56.4%. In the Brussels region, testing stood at 91.3% (4).

The "90-90-90 Goal" is the new 2016-2020 plan to combat TB, which aims to diagnose 90% of people with the disease, including 90% of the most vulnerable(pop) populations, and to ensure 90% treatment cures. If achieved, these goals should make it possible to eradicate the TB epidemic by 2035 (8).

Raising public awareness by upgrading people's knowledge and preventing this scourge seem to be among the most effective means of combating it. However, in the DRC, very few studies have been carried out on the subject. The study by AKETI et al in 2017 found that 92.6% of mothers had heard of TB, but only 44.2% knew that it was contagious and only 29.2% knew how it was transmitted.

The above shows that TB is little known among mothers. However, no study has been carried out among the general population in our area to determine their level of knowledge of this disease.

3. Objectives

- General objective:

  This study aims to contribute to the improvement of TB management in the city-province of Kinshasa by assessing the population's level of knowledge about this disease.

- Specific objectives:

- Describe the socio-economic characteristics of the population surveyed.
- Determine their level of knowledge of TB.
- Describe individual behavior in the face of TB.
- Compare this level of knowledge with the socio-economic conditions of the respondents.

CHAPTER 1. GENERAL INFORMATION

TB has existed for over 120 centuries. BK, the causative agent of TB, was discovered in the 19th century, in 1882. Once treated in sanatoria with sun and open-air cures, the incidence of TB declined in the 20th century, thanks to the development of hygiene and the appearance of the first antibiotics such as streptomycin in 1943. In 2013, an estimated 9 million people contracted the disease and 1.5 million died, including 360,000 HIV+ subjects. The disease is slowly receding each year, and an estimated 37 million lives were saved between 2000 and 2013 thanks to effective treatment and diagnosis (12). One of the new features of the epidemic is an increase in multi-resistant strains (9).

1.1. Definition

TB is an infection caused by mycobacteria of the MT complex, and can manifest itself as latent tuberculosis infection (LTI) or active TB (AT). LTI is the presence of tubercle bacilli within the body, without any manifestation of the disease. Carriers of LTI are by definition non-contagious and pose no risk to those around them. Active TB is the disease caused by the presence of tubercle bacilli inside the body. Depending on the site of infection, it is manifested by various signs and symptoms, radiological abnormalities and the presence of bacilli in sputum or other clinical specimens. It may or may not be contagious, depending on the site and certain conditions.

1.2. Epidemiology

TB is still a major scourge, and many children die from it around the world. On a global scale, the incidence rate has been falling since early 2006.

Although unevenly distributed throughout the world, it remains one of mankind's greatest scourges (10). The WHO estimates that, in 2002, there were 2 billion people infected with the tubercle bacillus, 8,800,000 NC, 4,000,000 cases of pulmonary TB with bacilloscopy + and more than 1,800,000 deaths per year. The estimated incidence of contagious TB is 63 per 100,000 inhabitants worldwide, while in sub-Saharan Africa it reaches 149 per 100,000 inhabitants, and in Madagascar 77 per 100,000 inhabitants. The WHO estimates that TB is on the increase worldwide: annual incidence was 8.8 million in 2002, with a forecast of 10 million in 2005 (including 5 million smear+ pulmonary TB) (11).

The proportion of tuberculosis patients co-infected with HIV in 2002 was 10% worldwide, and 30% in sub-Saharan Africa.

A distinction is made between low-prevalence countries, where the aim is to eliminate TB despite the current epidemiological revival, and high-prevalence countries (which include most developing countries), where the aim is to control the disease.

1.3. Factors in progression to TB disease

In 1997, the WHO estimated that 7.96 million CKDs occurred worldwide, more than half of them contagious, and the majority (95%) occurred in the poorest countries due to inadequate health coverage (only 30% to 60% of these patients are detected and treated). (12)

The persistence of TB throughout the world and in Africa is also linked to poverty (95% of TB sufferers live in poor countries), population growth (over 6 billion in 2000; 7.9 billion forecast for 2025) and human migration.

Medical and social staff and people working with these at-risk groups account for around 2.7% (14). In the literature, there are classically medical situations that favor progression to "disease" TB: immunosuppression, with HIV-positive patients having a tuberculin + test, AIDS patients, organ transplant patients with drug-induced immunosuppression, patients receiving Anti-TNF drugs, corticosteroid therapy (more than 15 mg prednisolone equivalent per day for a period of more than 2 to 4 weeks), cancers (especially hematological malignancies, head and neck and lung tumors), chronic IR and hemodialysis, DS, smoking, alcoholism, age under 5 years, and other pathologies such as gastrectomies, jejuno-ileostomies and anthracosilicosis (12).

Until the 1980s, TB declined steadily in high-income countries. The first so-called "natural" decline occurred with the rise in people's standard of living before the era of chemotherapy; it then accelerated with the advent of specific antibiotics(AB) to reach figures close to elimination in countries that had set up highly effective control programs. The reversal of the downward trend was noted as early as 1979 in the major cities of the United States, with the greatest increases recorded in New York City. This was particularly true of people under 45, blacks, Hispanics and migrants from Asia and the Pacific. In 1993, this increase ceased, except for cases reported in children under fifteen (Tx. in native children are higher. They are 18.8 per 100,000 for children under 5 and 9.8 per 100,000 for children aged 5 to 14).

This increase was accompanied by high mortality, but especially among 20 to 49 year-olds in states with large urban populations, where there was a high proportion of both HIV-infected subjects and poor or homeless people. This phenomenon was subsequently observed in a large number of Western and Eastern European countries, particularly in large cities.

The recent resurgence of TB in high-income countries is linked to the social marginalization of disadvantaged groups, the onset of the HIV epidemic, the dismantling of anti-TB structures and migration from countries with a high proportion of TB-infected subjects.

This phenomenon is also found in European capitals, where the ratio of incidence to the rest of the country, in 2009, showed Brussels 3.1; London 3; Paris 2.9; Copenhagen 2.8; Oslo 2.8; Rome 2.8; Amsterdam 2.7 (13). With Europe's migration crisis, the incidence of TB in major cities is set to rise. In 1991 in Belgium, 18% of TB patients were non-Belgian, compared with 52% in 2013.

1.4. Pathogenesis and transmission

Transmission is by inhalation of aerosols (airborne), with human-to-human contamination from droplets of aerosolized respiratory secretions. This occurs in TB with pulmonary or laryngeal involvement. The risk of transmission depends on the degree of contagiousness (direct or indirect) of the case, the type of contact (duration, proximity), the immune vulnerability of exposed persons (children under 5, HIV and immunocompromised people) and the environment (ventilation, natural light). In general, the longer the exposure, the greater the risk of transmission. After contact with a patient presenting with pulmonary TB, 30 to 65% of patients will be contaminated (15).

For pulmonary or laryngeal TB, the contagious period lasts as long as the infected person excretes tubercle bacilli in sputum. It diminishes rapidly after the start of effective treatment. Children under the age of 10 suffering from pulmonary TB are generally considered not very contagious, as lesions are minimal, bacilli excretion is negligible and coughing is generally absent.

LTI is not contagious. Extra-pulmonary forms of TB are not contagious, except in exceptional situations.

Once contracted, BK multiplies in pulmonary macrophages. After an incubation period of 6 to 8 weeks, BK invades the lymphatic tract, hilar lymph nodes and bloodstream. The body reacts by developing cellular immunity, leading to spontaneous recovery within six months in 90-95% of patients: this is known as the latent primary infection state. Progression to TB reactivation within two years will be around 2%, depending on the risk factors discussed above. A small percentage (just 5-10%) will progress to "disease" TB (patent primary infection) within two years, and this will depend on the patient's age, mycobacterial load and underlying immune status (15). In children, the risk of primary TB and extra-pulmonary forms (miliary and neuro-meningeal) is high. It is particularly high in children under 5 years of age. Adolescents are more at risk of developing classic pulmonary TB (16). The intensity of the mycobacterial load is also important for the progression to "disease" TB. A TB patient with direct examination - and culture + will have an intradermoreaction (IDR) conversion Tx. of 25.7% and a progression to TA of 5.7%, whereas one with direct examination + and culture + will have a much higher IDR conversion Tx. (66%) and a progression to TA of 35.6% (16). Underlying immunodeficiency will also play a role: 40% of HIV-infected children will progress to "disease" TB within 40 days. In the classical model, in summary, progression to either LTI or "disease" TB will depend on the patient's age and state of immunodepression, as well as the infectious load. In HIV patients, 30 to 40% will progress early to TB, whereas in normal people, 98% will be latent. Reactivation of the disease will be in the order of 2 to 10% in the normal population, compared with 20 to 50% in HIV patients. It is therefore important to remember that the classic model which divides TB into TA and ITL is much more complex than that, involving a continuum from latency to TA. There is evidence to suggest that, in this dynamic model, the spectrum ranges from dormant to fulminant, passing through a whole series of intermediate states, including miliary, extra pulmonary, pulmonary and chronic TB. Each state will depend on the bacterial load present, the state of immunosuppression, age, and then on the balance between pro- and anti-inflammatory action within the granulomas (17). One of the difficulties lies in distinguishing between reactivation and reinfection. A Dutch cohort showed that only 0.8% of migrant patients developed TB 15 years after arrival in a low-incidence territory. This suggests that reactivation is probably less frequent than reinfection (17).

1.5. Clinical charts

5.1. Latent TB

TB infection results from the first penetration of MT into an organism free from any previous contact. In 90% of cases, primary TB infection is clinically inapparent, with the bacillus remaining in a quiescent state. Subjects then present a latent TB. Latent infection (LTI), and may develop TB disease over the long term, either through exogenous reinfection (notion of contact) or endogenous reinfection (no notion of contact, due to poor hygiene, overwork, lack of sleep, lack of food and alcoholism having weakened immunity).

It is usually manifested by a reaction to the tuberculin skin test or PPD (TCT), or to the gamma interferon release test (TLIG). Infection will remain asymptomatic in 50% of children under 1 year of age, in 70-80% of children aged 1 to 2 and in 95-98% of children aged 2 to 10. In children over 10 years of age, 80-90% of infected children will not develop the disease.

5.2. Active TB

TA or TB disease is due to the bronchial dissemination of MT maintained until then by the primary lesions, such as healed caverns and primary infection lymph nodes. It is a source of transmission to close contacts. It accounts for 70% of TB cases worldwide. It can affect all body tissues by lymphatic or hematogenous route, in particular lymph nodes, bones, pleura, meninges and the urogenital tract. A distinction is made between pulmonary and extrapulmonary TB.

Pulmonary TB was the most frequent form (70-75% of cases), compared with 30% for extrapulmonary TB and 8.5% for mixed forms (14).

Tb can present in a classic form: lesions located mainly in the upper lobes and posterior segments, or in the form of miliaria, which is a dissemination of TB throughout the body.

There is also a pleural form with pleural effusion. The last pulmonary form is tuberculous pneumonia, linked to the massive seeding of BK in healthy parenchyma from an excavated lesion associated with an intense inflammatory reaction resembling community-acquired pneumonia (15).

The extrapulmonary forms (50%) are lymph node and osteoarticular involvement is the second most common, mainly in the spinal region or mal de Pott (15), as well as meningeal, genital, renal and bladder forms.

Symptoms:

Symptoms are typically dominated by fever or febrile spells, nocturnal sweating, weight loss, fatigue and inappetence.

Symptoms are directly related to their location, e.g. in the lung, coughing, hemoptoic sputum, dyspnea and chest discomfort. In extra-pulmonary TB, symptoms are dominated, for example, by back pain or weakness in the legs when the spinal cord is involved. Meningeal TB, on the other hand, may present with altered general condition, headaches and a meningeal picture (15). The extra-pulmonary form is named after the organ affected (renal, bone or meningeal TB, or tuberculous adenitis).

The deeper the immunodepression, the more likely it is that non-cavitary, extra-pulmonary and, above all, disseminated forms will appear (15).

1.6. Paraclinical examinations

Paraclinical tests are divided into BK detection tests and referral tests. With regard to the first group, these tests are now compulsory as part of the diagnostic process, even if the result is still not positive. They include

- examination of the sample under a microscope (3x for sputum),
- cultivation, which is particularly time-consuming (6 weeks on average),
- molecular methods, which are in full expansion, and,
- histology (GenXpert, PCR, etc.).

Referral examinations include tests that demonstrate recent contact with BK and medical imaging that serve as a guide. This group includes

- TCT and TLIG (these tests are used to detect ITL),
- radiology (including X-rays of the thorax or other relevant organs, CT scans, bronchoscopy, etc.). These examinations are particularly revealing in adults, often with classic cavitary pneumonia, and in children and adolescents, in whom the radiological picture mainly shows mediastinal and hilar adenopathies, sometimes accompanied by parenchymal infiltrates.

Direct examination is not always + (In Belgium, only 44.4% of pulmonary TB cases had a + direct examination, while culture was + in 78.2% of all reported TB cases and in 84.9% of pulmonary TB cases). Hence the importance of molecular techniques, in particular GenXpert (these new, much more powerful techniques not only enable us to have a rapid response to the diagnosis (between 2 and 24 hours) but also detect sensitivity to rifampicin and isoniazid (INH) at the same time) (16). On lung samples, sensitivity is around 89% and specificity 99% (16). Sensitivity varies according to whether direct examination is + or -. When direct examination is +, sensitivity is of the order of 98%, and when direct examination is -, sensitivity is of the order of 75% (16). Sensitivity also varies according to the type of extra-lung specimen. We know, for example, that GenXpert has a good sensitivity of around 85% for central nervous system samples, and 97% for lymph node samples. Results are poor for pleural fluid, with a sensitivity of around 37%. The other fluids, peritoneal and pericardial, are found with a sensitivity of around 67%. Gastric fluid has a sensitivity of around 80%. Specificity is extremely good, ranging from 93% to 99% (17). In 2013, the WHO issued recommendations for the diagnosis of TB. It points out that the predictive value of GenXpert is low, particularly in low-prevalence countries. Culture remains indispensable in all cases (18). For the diagnosis of rifampin resistance, the predictive value - is greater than 99% in both high- and low-prevalence countries. The + predictive value is highly dependent on prevalence. In high-prevalence countries, and in patients already treated, it is 99%, whereas in low-prevalence countries, it is less than 70%, hence the possibility of a second GenXpert test. The WHO clearly recommends GenXpert as a first-line test for pulmonary forms in adults and children suspected of having multidrug-resistant TB or HIV-associated TB (strong recommendation), and when direct examination is - in low-risk populations with multidrug-resistant TB or HIV (weak recommendation). In extra-pulmonary forms, the WHO recommends its use in the diagnosis of meningeal forms, the advantage being a much more rapid diagnosis (strong recommendation). The recommendation is intermediate for lymph node forms (18). Clearly, GenXpert should not be used to monitor treatment. The development of molecular techniques, in particular GenXpert, has made it possible not only to make a much more rapid diagnosis, with relatively good sensitivity and specificity, depending on the type of sample, but also to rapidly detect any resistance to rifampicin and INH (16-18).

1.7. Multidrug-resistant TB

Table 5. Clinical criteria leading to suspicion of multidrug-resistant TB (MDR-TB) (19)

History of previous treatment
- Poor compliance
- Multiple side effects
- Absorption disorders
Originating from or travelling to a country with a high prevalence of MDR-Tb
Contact with a patient with MDR-TB
Treatment failure of a well-conducted first-line ANTI-T therapy

Monoresistance refers to resistance to one first-line treatment agent. Polyresistance occurs when the TM is resistant to two or more first-line agents other than INH or rifampin. Multidrug resistance (MDR) refers to resistance to both rifampicin and INH. Extensive multidrug resistance (XDR) occurs when the MT is resistant to INH and rifampicin, and to any quinolone and another second-line treatment agent. Pre-extensive multidrug resistance (Pre-XDR) is defined as resistance to rifampin and INH, and resistance to fluoroquinolones or second-line agents (Table 3). Another definition is acquired multi-resistance, for patients who have been previously treated with ANTI-T therapy. Finally, primary multiresistance occurs when a patient has been infected through contact with a multiresistant germ.

Table 6. Resistance definition

Monoresistance	BK resistant to 1 First-line ANTI-T
Polyresistance	BK resistant to 2 or more first-line ANTI-Ts other than Rifampicin and INH
Multiresistance (MDR)	BK resistant to Rifampicin and INH
Extensive multiresistance (XDR)	BK resistant to Rifampicin and INH and to one of the quinolones and at least 1 of the second-line ANTI-Ts
Pre-XDR	BK resistant to Rifampicin and INH and to quinolones or to at least 1 of the second-line ANTI-Ts

1.8. The treatment

The first ABs were discovered in 1943. It was streptomycin (28).

It's important to point out that for at least 35 years, or even 45 years, TB treatment has changed little or not at all, with the exception of multidrug resistance. This treatment involves a combination of four first-line ANTI-T drugs: INH, rifampin, pyrazinamide and ethambutol (Table III). In general, quadritherapy is prescribed for 2 months, followed by dual therapy with rifampicin and INH for 4 months.

It's important to realize that, in this combination, the ABs play a different role, allowing us to understand the underlying reason for this combination of antibiotics.

- **Isoniaside (INH)** is a powerful bactericide, reducing the bacterial load by over 92% in two days. It is followed by rifampicin. It has some activity on bacilli in acidic pH (hydrogen potential), but virtually no activity in neutral pH, notably in caseous foci.

- **Pyrazinamide:** has very low bactericidal activity at the start of treatment. Pyrazinamide is mainly active against slowly multiplying bacilli at acid pH, i.e. macrophages, and has virtually no activity against slowly multiplying bacilli at neutral pH, in particular caseous foci.

  Rifampicin, on the other hand, is active at all three stages of multiplication.

- **Ethambutol:** has little effect on the different phases of growth, its main role being to prevent the selection of INH-resistant bacilli.

In short, INH is the major early bactericide, with 95% of the inoculum wiped out in two days (bactericidal effect from 18 mg/d, with an increasing effect up to 300 mg/d). Ethambutol, for its part, has a weak effect on the different phases of growth, its role being primarily to prevent the selection of INH-resistant bacilli. Pyrazinamide is most effective when INH-resistant strains are present (29).

Table 7. First-line ANTI-T

Medicines	Admini strati on quoti dienne			Administration intermittent 3x/Sem.		
	Children	Adults	Maximum dose mg/day	Children	Adults	Maximum dose mg/day
Isoniazid	5-10 (15)	5	300	10	10 (15)	900
Rifampicin	10-20	10	600	10	10	600
Pyrazinamide	25-40	25	2000	35-50	35	2.000
Ethambutol	15(25)*	15 (25)	1600	30	30	2.000

0 Increased dose for severe TB

25 mg no more than 30 days

N.B.: Withholding INH in TB treatment will result in less rapid sputum negativation; withholding rifampicin will extend treatment duration to 18 months; withholding pyrazinamide may extend treatment duration to 9 months (29).

The classic regimen consists of two months' quadritherapy (initial phase) with INH, rifampin, pyrazinamide and ethambutol, followed by 4 months' dual therapy (continuation phase) with INH and rifampin. There are intermittent regimens with an initial two-month phase and daily quadritherapy (INH, rifampin, pyrazinamide and ethambutol) and a continuation phase with 3x/week INH and rifampin (20). It is important to note that the intermittent regimen is only used in the maintenance phase and should not be applied in immunocompromised patients, particularly HIV patients (Table III).

The treatment of extra-pulmonary TB is identical to that of pulmonary TB, at least in terms of the combination regimen. Among additive drugs, we have pyridoxine, which is vitamin B6 (Vit B6) at a dose of 20 mg/d, 250 mg/week, to prevent peripheral neuropathy caused by INH. In practice, it is routinely administered , but it may not be. Its use is especially recommended for at-risk patients such as pregnant or breast-feeding women, alcoholics, the elderly, malnourished subjects, diabetics, renal failure sufferers, HIV-infected subjects and breast-fed children. During pregnancy, Vit B6 should be administered at a slightly higher dose of 25 mg/d. In pregnant women, vitamin K (Vit K) should be administered during the last two weeks of pregnancy, at a dose of 10 mg/d, and to the newborn at a dose of 1 mg/d, as there is a risk of haemorrhage. Breast-feeding women with tb should receive a full course of treatment with standard quadruple chemotherapy. Treatment must be rapid to prevent transmission of TB to the child. Mother and baby are often together, and the baby must continue to be breastfed, especially in developing countries. TB in children must be ruled out, and preventive treatment with INH must be given for 6 months, followed by BCG vaccination (20).

Corticoids are indicated for meningitis and pericarditis. In children, they can be used in tb miliary disease or in mediastinal lymph node forms causing compression with a reduction in bronchial diameter of more than 50%. Corticoids have also been used in immune restitution syndromes (IS) in patients on antiretroviral therapy (ART). When using cortisone, it should be remembered that it interacts with rifampicin, and it is advisable to increase the dose to 1.5 mg/kg/d (20).

Monitoring anti-TB treatment

The patient should be seen in consultation twice during the first month and once a month for up to a year post-diagnosis. Liver function tests, renal function tests, uricemia, complete blood count, CRP and HIV tests and visual function tests should be carried out at the start of treatment. Liver tests may be repeated at 15 days, 1st month and $2^{(nd)}$) month to monitor possible ANTI-T toxicity. Blood counts may be checked at month 2. Chest X-rays are taken on admission at 2th months and at the end of treatment. It may be checked at 12th months if there are any sequelae. Direct examination of sputum is carried out on admission, at 15 days. This examination, at 15 days, enables the patient to be discharged from quarantine on three occasions when he is -. It should also be carried out at 2th months. If it is positive at 2th month, it should be repeated at 3th month and, if it remains +, treatment failure should be discussed and the possibility of resistance raised. If the direct examination remains + at 5th months, the patient should be considered to have failed treatment, re-evaluated and treatment adaptation discussed in the light of any resistance found (20).

TB treatment must be taken extremely regularly. It is therefore essential to be vigilant. Direct administration techniques have been developed to help improve compliance.

Management of irregular intake or interruption of treatment will take into account the patient's situation: direct examination - or a culture + after interruption, interruption during the intensive phase rather than in the continuation phase, of long duration in the intensive phase (<2 sem or >2 sem), <2 months or >2 months in continuation phase, whether the interruption occurred early (before 4 months or after 4 months) in the continuation phase, whether the patient is immunosuppressed (particularly HIV) or has another immunosuppressive condition, whether the patient had a good or poor response to treatment before the interruption, and whether multidrug resistance is present or suspected. In the case of a sensitive tb, interruptions are managed as follows (Table 5). In the initial phase, if the interruption lasts less than two weeks, treatment should be extended to the duration initially planned; if the interruption lasts longer than two weeks, treatment should be restarted from the beginning. During the continuation phase, if the interruption lasts less than two months, treatment should be extended to reach the duration initially planned; if the interruption lasts more than two months, it should be checked whether the patient has taken his or her treatment regularly, and whether he or she has taken treatment for a total of at least 4 months. In this case, it will be necessary to complete the treatment to reach the duration initially planned. If the treatment has been taken irregularly, or for less than 4 months in total, the treatment should be restarted from the very beginning (20).

Another problem facing clinicians is the management of side-effects, in particular impaired liver function. In the presence of impaired hepatic function, it is important to check that the dose corresponds to the patient's weight, especially for pyrazinamide, which must be less than 25 mg/kg/day. Toxic causes other than anti-T therapy must be ruled out (alcohol, including any other hepatotoxic medications, must be eliminated). If there is a disturbance of enzymes only, and transaminases between 3 and 5 times normal, without a clinical picture of hepatitis, treatment should be continued and biological monitoring reinforced. If the transaminase disturbance is 5x higher than normal, with no clinical picture of hepatitis, not all anti-T drugs should be stopped, but the most hepatotoxic should be withdrawn first, notably INH and pyrazinamide, while rifampicin and ethambutol are maintained. INH is reintroduced, gradually increasing the dose; as soon as transaminases have returned to normal, or when transaminases are less than 2 times normal, pyrazinamide is added at a low dose (15-20 mg/kg). If transaminases remain disturbed, pyrazinamide should be discontinued. If the clinical picture is one of clinical hepatitis with jaundice and elevated bilirubin, all anti-T therapy should be stopped. As soon as there is clinical and biological improvement, standard treatment is gradually reintroduced, first ethambutol with rifampin, then INH. Any reintroduction of pyrazinamide must be discussed within the team. If the tb is severe and life-threatening, an alternative anti-T treatment with low hepatotoxicity should be prescribed: e.g. ethambutol + a fluoroquinolone + an aminoglycoside, until the standard treatment can be re-prescribed.

As a general rule, after complete discontinuation of ANTI-T therapy, rifampin (with or without ethambutol) is reintroduced as soon as transaminases have fallen to less than 2 x normal. After 3 to 7 days, INH can be reintroduced while transaminases are monitored. If symptoms reappear or transaminases rise, the last medication introduced should be discontinued. In patients who have suffered severe prolonged impairment of hepatotoxicity but who have tolerated the reintroduction of rifampin and INH well, however, the addition of pyrazinamide should be considered with caution. If it is decided to stop pyrazinamide for good, treatment should be extended to 9 months. In the case of IR or hemodialysis patients, the dose of first-line ANTI-Ts should be adapted for patients with glomerular filtration or creatinine clearance below 30 ml/min, or for patients receiving hemodialysis. INH and rifampicin do not require dose adjustment; however, pyrazinamide will be administered at 35 mg/kg 3x/week, while ethambutol will be administered at 15 to 25 mg/kg 3x/week (20).

Table 8. Regular or interrupted catch management

Time of interruption	Duration of interruption	Attitude
Initial phase	< 2 wks.	Extend the treatment to reach the originally planned duration
Initial phase	> 2 weeks	Start treatment from the beginning
Continuation phase	< 2 months	Extend the treatment to reach the originally planned duration
Continuation phase	> 2 months	If regular treatment taken for a total of at least 4 months, the treatment must be completed If irregular treatment or treatment taken for less than 4 months, the treatment must be restarted from the very beginning.

If rifampicin is unusable for tolerability reasons, a two-month regimen of isoniazid, ethambutol, pyrazinamide + moxifloxacin + 13 months of INH, ethambutol, moxifloxacin can be administered. A possible alternative to rifampicin is a classic regimen with rifabutin. If INH is unusable, due to resistance or tolerance, a six-month regimen with rifampicin, ethambutol and pirazinamide is possible. If pirazinamide is unusable, two months of isoniazid, rifampin and ethambutol + 7 months of INH and rifampin for a total of 9 months. If ethambutol is unusable, in the absence of resistance, there is no impact on treatment (20).

Duration of treatment

Treatment duration is 6 months for pulmonary and extra-pulmonary forms of TB, except for neuromeningeal forms, where it is 9 to 12 months. For osteoarticular forms, there is a debate between conventional 6-month treatment versus 9 to 12 months.

This may seem an extremely long time. It is therefore important to be able to look for new combinations or new molecules that can shorten this period. In this respect, the use of quinolones has proved to be a possible alternative. The first to be tried was the substitution of moxifloxacin for INH in the intensive phases of pulmonary TB treatment. Dorman et al were able to show that substitution of moxifloxacin for INH led to an increase in negative cultures at 8 weeks (30). This increase was modest but not statistically significant. In a randomized phase ii study using moxifloxacin as initial therapy for TB, Gonde et al (31) showed that it significantly increased negative culture response. This raised the question of whether quinolones could be used to reduce the duration of treatment. Several studies along these lines have recently been published (3234).

These alternative regimens initially used gatifloxacin with a 4-month regimen of rifampicin, isoniazid, pyrazinamide and gatifloxacin versus a conventional 6-month regimen with two months of rifampicin, isoniazid, pyrazinamide, ethambutol + 4 months of rifampicin and INH. This trial failed to show the non-inferiority of gatifloxacin in a 4-month regimen (32).

The second trial used moxifloxacin: 17 wks rifampicin, INH, pyrazinamide, moxifloxacin or 17 wks rifampicin, ethambutol, pyrazinamide, moxifloxacin versus 8 wks rifampicin, isoniazid, pyrazinamide, ethambutol and 18 wks rifampicin, isoniazid. Again, this trial did not show that the use of moxifloxacin shortened the treatment regimen compared with the conventional regimen (33).

A third regimen was the use of moxifloxacin plus rifapentine. We had a regimen comprising two months of rifampicin, moxifloxacin, pyrazinamide, ethambutol + 2 months of moxifloxacin and 900 mg rifapentine 2x/week or two months of rifampicin, moxifloxacin, pyrazinamide, ethambutol + 4 months moxifloxacin and 1200 mg rifabutin 1x/week versus a regimen with two months rifampicin, INH, pyrazinamide, ethambutol + 4 months rifampicin, isoniazid, pyrazinamide, ethambutol. This trial showed no non-inferiority for the 4-month regimen (34).

It's important to remember that these ANTI-T substances only act on young lesions, and not on old, poorly irrigated ones. As a result, while their use has greatly reduced mortality, it has not greatly reduced the number of chronic tuberculosis patients. This is why other treatments can either replace or complement this antibiotic therapy, and we quote:

- Chemotherapy,
- Radiotherapy,
- Surgery.

1.9. Prevention

TB prevention involves a number of factors:

1. Vaccination

   In 1921, Albert Calmette and Camille Guérin successfully tested the first vaccine against TB, which they named BACILLE CALMETTE GUERIN, or BCG for short. BCG vaccination is a primo-infection with a fixed, non-virulent germ, given at a chosen moment when the healthy subject reacts well and will benefit from immunity, which lasts several years but is only achieved after six semesters, during which time the child must live away from everyone, and therefore cannot prevent transmission of the disease and halt the worldwide epidemic.

2. Screening for carrier cattle:

   In order to prevent transmission of the bacillus to humans, either by direct contact via the air, or via the digestive tract following ingestion of undercooked or pasteurized meat or milk, the WHO has called for all cattle herds to be sanitized since 2000. This preventive measure is based on the fight against indirect contagion.

3. Social measures:

   TB, a social disease, finds much of its proliferation in the considerable influence of lack of ventilation and sunlight, lack of property too often accompanied by bad food, smoking and alcoholism.

   Within a given city, TB is most prevalent in poor, overcrowded neighborhoods, where it respects even the most salubrious homes.

   These preventive measures include

a) Improving the terrain:

- The development of personal hygiene;
- The outdoor life;
- The physical culture;
- The general cleanliness;
- The food;
- Sufficient and regular sleep; etc...

-Social measures proper:

- Destruction of unhealthy areas;
- Creation of wide streets, large open spaces;
- Stop overcrowding in cities and build comfortable, healthy homes;
- Improving working conditions in certain professions, home education for mothers and even the whole population, combating alcoholism and smoking;
- Radiology for early detection of primary infection to facilitate treatment. **b)** Contagion control

It will include a whole range of measures:

- No spitting on the ground, on trains or bus stops... (dispose of feeders and personal objects)
- Frequent disinfection of public premises;
- Screening in communities (schools, camps, administration, etc.) for the sick and predisposed;
- Managing HIV cases to reduce their impact on TB. (31)

c) Isolation

It's important to remember that the degree to which TB is contagious can be estimated from the positivity of the various microbiological tests that assess the bacterial load. The greater the bacterial load, the more contagious the disease. Positive direct examination is superior to PCR, which in turn is superior to culture +. All contagious patients should be kept in respiratory isolation until three sputum samples taken one day apart have been - on direct microscopic examination. When the initial direct examination obtained after gastric lavage is +, the decision to discontinue isolation will be based on the result of a new gastric sampling. In the case of a patient whose bronchoalveolar lavage is + on initial direct examination, discontinuation of isolation will be decided on the basis of the patient's radio-clinical evolution and the disappearance of the cough. In principle, bronchoalveolar lavage is not repeated. If resistance is suspected, isolation should be maintained until antibiotic susceptibility testing has confirmed the bacilli's sensitivity to first-line anti-T drugs (20). At present, PCR provides a rapid indication of resistance to rifampicin or INH (26).

CHAPTER 2. MATERIALS AND METHODS

2.1. Equipment

- Study framework

Our study took place in the city and province of Kinshasa, in the four districts of randomly selected churches: the Communauté Batiste au Congo (CBCO) in Bandal 1 for FUNA, the Kitambo French-speaking CBCO for LUKUNGA, the Saint Augustin LEMBA church for MONT AMBA, and the réveille toi qui dort church for TSHANGU.

- Study period

It ran for one month, from April 01 to April 30, 2019.

- Study population

It involved all adult men and women living in the provincial city of Kinshasa, whether or not they had contracted TB.

- Sampling

- Inclusion criteria: any person aged 18 or over who has given informed consent.
- Non-inclusion criteria: any non-adult, i.e. under 18, and any adult without consent.
- Sample size and rationale: The sample size was set at 300. The choice of churches was random: we randomly selected a church in each health district of the city of Kinshasa, after listing the most frequented churches. We opted for a survey in the churches because of their representativeness, since all social strata are found in the churches.

- Materials used for collection

- A survey form has been drawn up, entered and multiplied to record the data collected from the population;
- A pen.

2.2 Methods

- Type of study.

This is a cross-sectional survey.

- Data collection procedure

After obtaining permission from the church committee, we proceeded to train the survey team (health staff and other trained people), a brief presentation by the pastor to the congregation and then the actual data collection.

- Parameters of interest
- socio-demographic parameters
- socio-economic parameters
- clinical variables
- knowledge of TB and the BCG vaccine
- Operational definitions

- Socioeconomic level(NSE): was defined by a score considering the assets owned by the respondent and housing characteristics according to EDS 2014. Socioeconomic level will be considered:

  ✓ low economic level: 0-3

  ✓ medium: from 4-8

  ✓ high: >9.

❖ Level of knowledge about TB: was assessed on the basis of knowledge about means of prevention, the definition of TB and the mode of transmission.

  ❖ No knowledge: score = nil

  ❖ Low knowledge: score =1

  ❖ Average knowledge: score = 2

  ❖ High knowledge: score = 3

❖ Good knowledge: of at least the definition of TB, means of prevention and mode of transmission.

- Large households are those with more than 6 people, according to MICS RDC-2010.

- Data analysis

Once the data had been encoded and validated, they were entered on the computer, using Microsoft Excel 2010 software. Systematic cleaning of the file was carried out using the completeness test and the consistency test, in order to harmonize and validate the data. Once the database was complete, analyses were carried out using SPSS 22 software. The statistics used to describe the variables were mean ± standard deviation for quantitative variables. Qualitative variables were described in terms of relative frequency (%) and/or absolute frequency (n).

Proportions were compared using the chi-square test for categorical data, and means were compared using Student's t-test.

- Ethical considerations

Authorization from the Faculty of Medicine and the Department of Pediatrics was obtained before the study began.

The authorization of the committee of the various churches (namely the Communauté Batiste au Congo(CBCO) de Bandal 1 for the FUNA, the Kitambo francophone CBCO for the LUKUNGA, in the Saint Augustin LEMBA church for the MONT AMBA and finally in the réveille toi qui dort church for the TSHANGU) was also obtained before any data collection.

Informed consent was obtained from the respondents before data collection began.

The questionnaires were anonymous and used only by the survey team to maintain confidentiality.

CHAPTER 3. RESULTS

3.1. Socio-demographic characteristics

Table 5. Socio-demographic characteristics of the study population

Variables	Numbers (n=300)	Percentage
Age		
<20 years	52	17,3
21-30 years old	147	49,0
31-40 years	47	15,7
41-50 years	29	9,7
>50 years	25	8,3
Gender		
Male	140	46,7
Female	160	53,3
Profession		
Civil servant	99	33,0
Liberal	38	12,7
unemployed	47	15,7
Student	116	38,7
Religion		
Catholic	95	31,7
Protestant	92	30,7
Eglise de Réveil	95	31,7
Kimbanguist	18	6,0
Study level		
No	7	2,3
Primary	14	4,7
Secondary	77	25,7
University	202	67,3

Socio-demographic characteristics are summarized in Table 5, which shows that the majority of respondents were aged between 21-30 years (49%). Their average age was 30.4±11.9 years, with extremes ranging from 18 to 81 years. Women were more represented with 53.3% and a sex ratio F/H of 1.2. The majority of civil servants answered our questions (33%). Catholic and revivalist believers were the most numerous (31.7% respectively). Respondents were more likely to be university graduates.

Table 6. Socio-familial characteristics of the study population

Variables	Numbers (n=300)	Percentage
Number of children		
No	201	67,0
1-5	78	26,0
>6	21	7,0
Household size		
1-6	190	63,3
>7	110	36,7
NSE		
Bottom	136	45,3
Medium	144	48,0
High	20	6,7

This table shows that more than half the respondents had no children (67%), the majority of households surveyed had fewer than 6 people, and 48% had an average socio-economic level, while 45% had a low one.

3.2. Knowledge of TB

3.2.1. Overall level of knowledge about TB

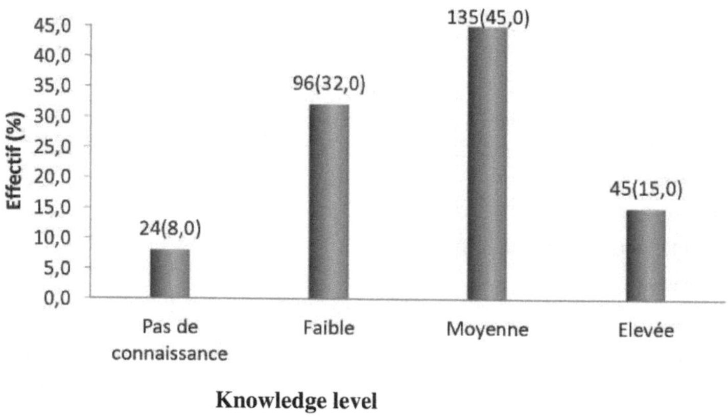

Figure 1: Respondents' overall level of knowledge about TB

Figure 1 shows that the majority of respondents had an average level of knowledge (45%), with only 15% having a high level of knowledge of TB.

3.2.2. Specific knowledge

3.2.2.1. TB information and information media

All respondents were already informed about TB. The means of information about TB are summarized in the figure below.

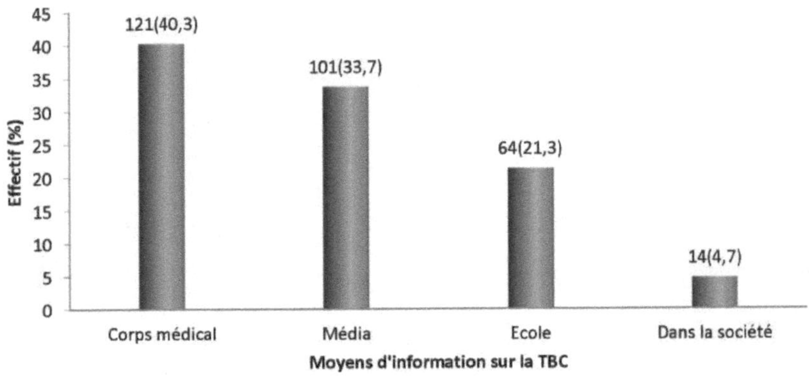

Figure 2: Distribution of TB information resources

The majority of respondents had been informed about TB by a medical body (40.3%) and through the media (33.7%).

3.2.2.2. Definition of TB

Table 7. Distribution of respondents according to TB definition

Definition of TB	Workforce	Percentage
Lung disease	106	35,3
Cough disease	63	21,0
Chronic, contagious and infectious disease	61	20,3
Smokers' disease	29	9,7
Don't know	25	8,3
Contagious disease transmitted by Bacillus Koch	16	5,3
Total	300	100,0

The majority of respondents defined TB as a lung disease (35.3%) and cough disease (21%). Only 5.3% defined TB as a contagious disease transmitted by BK.

3.2.2.3. Knowledge of mode of transmission and contagiousness

Table 8. Respondents' knowledge of mode of transmission and contagiousness

Variables	Numbers (n=300)	Percentage
Indirect transmission mode		
Contage 1st degree	162	54,0
Contage 2nd degree	20	6,7
Dust	18	6,0
Don't know	100	33,3
Direct transmission mode		
Through respiratory secretions	242	80,7
Unprotected food	11	3,7
Using the objects of tuberculosis patients	25	8,3
Don't know	22	7,3
Contagious disease No	8	2,7
Yes	292	97,3

Among the indirect modes of transmission, 54% recognized that TB is transmitted by 1st degree contagion and 33.3% didn't know. On the other hand, 80.7% of respondents recognized that TB is transmitted directly by respiratory secretions and 97.3% knew that TB is a contagious disease.

3.2.2.4. Knowledge of TB signs

Table 9. Knowledge of TB signs

Variables	Numbers (n=300)	Percentage
Suspected signs of TB		
Cough	274	91,3
Profound weight loss	94	31,3
Dyspnea	13	4,3
Diarrhea	4	1,3
Clinical signs of TB		
Oily cough	260	86,7
Weight loss	119	39,7
Fever	86	28,7
Anorexia	43	14,3
Asthenia	33	11,0
Profuse sweating	27	9,0

Cough (91.3%) and weight loss (31.3%) were the signs of suspected TB recognized by respondents. In contrast, the clinical signs of TB recognized by respondents were cough (86.7%), weight loss (39.7%) and fever (28.7%).

3.2.2.5. Knowledge of TB diagnostics

Table 10. Respondents' knowledge of TB diagnostics

Knowledge	**Numbers (n=300)**	**Percentage**
Examination of sputum	279	93,0
Chest X-ray	53	17,7
Blood test	10	3,3
Gen Xpert	0	0,0
Culture	0	0,0

This table shows that the majority of respondents recognize sputum examination as a means of diagnosing TB (93%).

3.2.2.6. Treatment knowledge

Table 11. Respondents' knowledge of TB treatment

Variables	**Workforce**	**Percentage**
In hospital by Anti-T	204	68,0
With TBAs	37	12,3
By Anti-T + ATB	33	11,0
Don't know	22	7,3
With traditional products	4	1,3
Total	300	100,0

This table shows that 68% of respondents were aware that TB is treated in hospital with anti-T drugs.

3.2.2.7. Knowledge of prevention methods

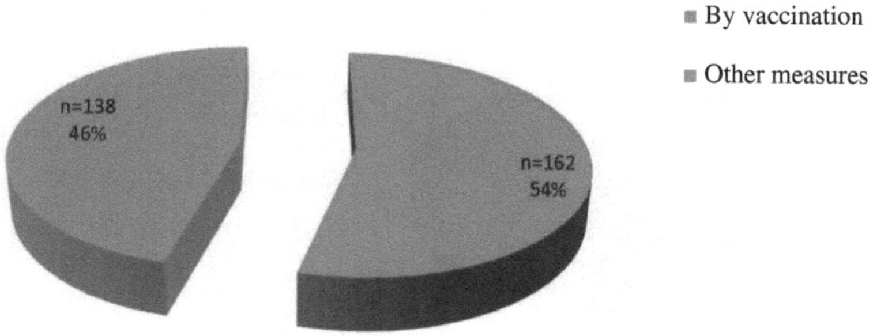

Figure 3: Knowledge of prevention methods

Vaccination is known as a means of preventing TB in 54% of respondents.

3.2.2.6. Knowledge of vaccination

Table 12. Respondents' knowledge of vaccination

Variables	Numbers (n=300)	Percentage
BCG vaccine knowledge		
Yes	127	42,3
No	173	57,7
Age of BCG administration		
0-9 months	20	6,7
10 months-12 years	41	13,7
at birth	79	26,3
Don't know	160	53,3
Knowledge of the vaccination record		
Yes	80	26,7
No	220	73,3

BCG vaccination was known by 42.3% of respondents; the majority of respondents did not know the age at which BCG is administered (53.3%), and only 26.3% knew that BCG vaccination is given at birth.

3.3. Attitude to TB

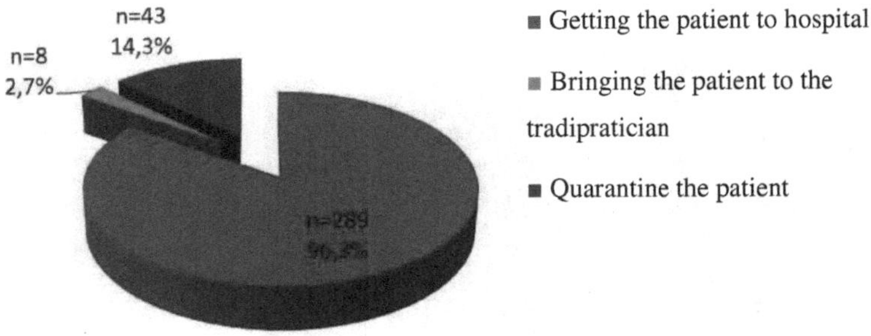

Figure 4. Respondents' attitudes to TB

When faced with TB, the majority of respondents adopt the attitude of taking the patient to hospital (96.3%), while 2.7% take the TB patient to a traditherapist.

3.4. Knowledge of TB and socio-demographic characteristics

The characteristics of respondents with good and poor knowledge of TB were comparable. Except for occupation, where civil servants had a higher frequency of good knowledge (p=0.048), and religion, where Protestants and Kimbanguists had a higher frequency of good knowledge about TB (p=0.007).

Table 13. Knowledge of TB and socio-demographic characteristics

Variables	Knowledge of TB		p-value
	Good (n=45)	Poor (n=255)	
Age	31,8±11,4	30,2±12,0	0,210
<30 years	28(62,3)	61(67,0)	
31-50 years	11(24,4)	65(25,5)	
>50 years	6(13,3)	19(7,5)	
Gender			0,209
Male	24(53,3)	116(45,5)	
Female	21(46,7)	139(54,5)	
Profession			**0,048**
Civil servant	23(51,1)	76(29,8)	
Liberal	4(8,9)	34(13,3)	
Unemployed	5(11,1)	42(16,5)	
Student	13(28,9)	103(40,4)	
Number of children			0,802
No	30(66,7)	171(67,1)	
1-5	11(24,4)	67(26,3)	
>6	4(8,9)	17(6,7)	
Religion			**0,007**
Catholic	9(20,0)	86(33,7)	
Protestant	16(35,6)	76(29,8)	
Eglise de Réveil	12(26,7)	83(32,5)	
Kimbanguist	8(17,8)	10(3,9)	
Education level			0,071
Bottom	10(22,2)	88(35,5)	
High	35(77,8)	167(65,5)	
Household size			0,372
1-6	30(66,7)	160(62,7)	
>7	15(33,3)	95(37,3)	
NSE			0,346
Bottom	16(35,6)	120(47,1)	
Medium	25(55,6)	119(46,7)	
High	4(8,9)	16(6,3)	

CHAPTER 4. DISCUSSION

4.1. Socio-demographic characteristics

Gender

Women accounted for just over half (53.3%) of all study respondents, giving an F/H sex ratio of 1.2. A clearer female predominance was reported by Diarra in Mali, who reported an F/H sex ratio of 2.5 in the general population of Bamako [32]. This near-equality between men and women in our study could be explained by the fact that it involved all members of the selected churches, where men and women are almost in perfect equality.

Age

The 21-30 age group was the most represented among the study's respondents (49%). The same observation was made by Podeme in the DRC, who reported a rate of 77% for the same age group [33]. The predominance of this age group could be due to the fact that the majority of the DRC's population is made up of young people, more than 50% according to the EDS 2014 [34]. To this end, Ouedraogo M. et al. reported that the response rate in the city of Ouagadougou, during their survey, was higher in the 25 to 44 age group [35].

Education level

The majority of respondents were university graduates (67.3%). Ottmani et al. made a similar finding, reporting in their series a clear predominance of university graduates (54%) versus 46% of low-school graduates in urban Morocco [36]. The predominance of university graduates could be due to the fact that more educated people attend church, and the survey was carried out on Sundays when this category of people are not at work and are available to answer our questions. However, our result contradicts that of Deribew et al. in Ethiopia, who reported in their series a rate of 61.7% of non-educated people [37]. This difference can be explained by the different methods used in the two studies.

Socioeconomic level

Respondents from medium and low socio-economic backgrounds were in the majority in this study, a result justified by the high level of poverty in the population, the lack of work and the high unemployment rate, which prevents them from earning a satisfactory income to meet their household needs.

4.2. General knowledge of TB

Source of information on TB

All the respondents who took part in the study had already heard of TB. The medical profession and the media were their main sources of information in 40% and 33.7% of cases respectively. This could be explained by the fact that the majority of the study population frequent hospitals, where the term is increasingly discussed, and that television and radio stations are very accessible in the city of Kinshasa, sometimes even broadcasting in local languages. In Mali, Diarra found that radio broadcasting was the main means of information on TB for 45% of the population of Bamako. This was also the case for Portero in the Philippines, with 78.6% [38].

Overall knowledge of TB

At the end of this study, we can state that the population of Kinshasa had low knowledge of TB: 45% of people had average knowledge, 32% low knowledge, 8% no knowledge and 15% good knowledge of TB. These results differ from those of H. Zaher and colleagues [39], who found 37.5% low, 38.3% average and 24.2% good knowledge respectively in 1997 in Egypt, and Rita L. and colleagues [40], who found 66% good knowledge among Latin Americans in 2000. Knowledge was higher among civil servants and respondents from Protestant and Kimbanguist churches. The generally low level of knowledge about TB could be explained by the lack of information about TB at grassroots level, both in the community and in health care centers. This could be due to the fact that health-care staff, who play a key role in raising awareness in health-care facilities, are not always well informed about TB when they leave their training schools. This situation is confirmed by Ouedraogo's study, carried out in Burkina Faso in 2008, which found that medical students were unfamiliar with TB control policy [40]. Thus, a reform of TB teaching in training schools to adapt it to the immediate requirements of future agents is desirable. Added to this is the need to intensify TB awareness at grassroots level, involving community associations.

Specific knowledge of TB

Although the majority of the study population had heard of TB, few defined it correctly. The correct definition was found in 5.3% of respondents. This shows that, despite their level of education, respondents have too little interest in TB.

Concerning knowledge of the signs, mode of transmission and contagiousness of TB, a good number of respondents (around 87%) had a good knowledge of the main symptom of TB, the cough. 97.3% knew that TB was contagious, and 80.7% knew that respiratory secretions were the main means of transmission. Our figures are close to those reported by Maria et al [41] in the Philippines (62.9%; 96.8%; 85.4% respectively) and Deribew et al in Ethiopia (78.7%; 100%; 91.2% respectively) [37]. The successful integration of these important features of TB is indicative of the efforts made by the various anti-T programs, through their awareness-raising activities via the media, posters and the organization of education campaigns on World TB Day.

However, knowledge of certain modes of TB transmission was limited. Indeed, 12% of respondents indicated that eating or using objects belonging to TB patients could transmit TB. In Pakistan, Mushtaq et al [42] made the same observation. Dust as a mode of TB transmission was cited by 6% of respondents. These gaps in knowledge of modes of transmission may lead respondents to adopt unjustified behavior towards TB patients.

Regarding TB treatment, a good number of respondents were aware that TB is treated in hospital with anti-T drugs (68%). Our figures are close to those reported by MUSHTAQ in Pakistan and Diarra in Mali, who noted 62% knowledge of treatment and 34% knowledge of anti-T drugs respectively. The higher level of knowledge noted in our study could be explained by the fact that respondents have greater access to medical information on TB management.

However, the study also found that some respondents would turn to non-medical treatments for chronic coughs. These included traditional treatment (1.3% of respondents) and non-specific antibiotic therapy (12.3% of respondents). These attitudes appear to be linked, on the one hand, to the socio-cultural considerations these people have about TB, and, on the other, to the lack of a prompt response from healthcare staff to refer patients with a persistent chronic cough that does not respond to specific treatment. As a result, diagnosis and treatment are delayed [43].

The existence of a TB vaccine was known by only 42.3% of respondents. Our results are close to those found by Podeme in Congo (77%) and Mushtaq et al. in Pakistan (urban 43.8%, rural 32.7%). The low level of knowledge in our study could be due to a lack of information on the vaccines of the Expanded Program on Immunization (EPI), which should not be the sole preserve of health personnel.

CONCLUSION

Our study involved 300 adult respondents of relatively young age, with a slight female predominance. It showed that respondents had insufficient knowledge of TB. The gaps in knowledge concerned several important aspects of the disease, such as its occurrence in our regions, modes of contamination, treatment requirements and means of prevention.

However, there was a good knowledge of TB symptoms and contagiousness. Health institutions and the media (radio and television) were the main sources of information for the target group, and it was above all profession and religion that had the greatest influence on knowledge of the disease.

It is therefore necessary to improve the population's level of knowledge about TB if we are to contribute to the reduction of its transmission, the morbidity and mortality associated with it, and to its elimination.

RECOMMENDATIONS

- To the Congolese government
  - Include non-communicable diseases, particularly TB, in its millennium priorities by funding awareness campaigns.
  - carrier screening
  - Destruction of unhealthy areas;
  - Creation of wide streets, large open spaces;
  - Stop overcrowding in cities and build comfortable, healthy homes;
- To healthcare personnel
  - Raise awareness of TB, particularly among people with low socioeconomic status.
- To the general population
  - Get tested for TB;
  - Learn more about TB to avoid complications;
  - Adopt appropriate measures to limit the spread of this disease:
  - Improving the terrain:
  - The development of personal hygiene;
  - Life in the great outdoors;
  - General cleanliness;
  - Ownership of food;
  - Sufficient and regular sleep; etc...
  - Improving working conditions in certain professions, home education for mothers and even the whole population, combating alcoholism and smoking;
  - Radiology for early detection of primary infection to facilitate management.
  - Contagion control

- No spitting on the ground, on trains or bus stops... (dispose of feeders and personal objects)
- Frequent disinfection of public premises;
- Screening in communities (schools, camps, administration, etc.) for the sick and predisposed;
- Managing HIV cases to reduce their impact on TB. (31)
- Isolation

REFERENCES

1. Tropical Medicine, TB/centre René la busquière/université de Bordeaux/France.
2. European Centre for Disease Prevention and Control/ WHO Regional Office for Europe. TBs surveillance and monitoring in Europe 2015.
3. Belgian tuberculosis register 2013, FAReS asbl, March 2015.
4. (Global tuberculosis control/htm/TB/2005.349).
5. (Corbet et al 2003).
6. Global tuberculosis report 2000. WHO
7. Global tuberculosis report 2011. WHO
8. Global tuberculosis report 2015. WHO
9. Prasad R. Multidrug and extensively drug-resistant TB (M/XDR-TB): problems and solutions. Indian J Tuberc 2010 Oct; 57(4):180-91.
10. Ma Z, Lienhardt C, Mcilleron H, Nunn AJ, Wang x. Global tuberculosis drug development pipeline: the need and the reality. Lancet 2010 Jun 12; 375 (9731):2100-9.
11. La Fréquence de la TB pulmonaire en milieu carcéral de Bamako (Katzelma.T.W Bedah thèse de Pharmacie).
12. Solovic i1, Sester M, Gomez-Reino JJ, Rieder Hl, ehlers S, Milburn HJ, et al. The risk of tuberculosis related to tumour necrosis factor antagonist therapies: a TBNeT consensus statement. Eur Respir J 2010 Nov; 36(5):1185206. doi: 10.1183/09031936.00028510. epub 2010 Jun 7
13. Van Hest NA, Aldridge Rw, de Vries G, Sandgren A, Hauer B, Hayward A, et al. Tuberculosis control in big cities and urban risk groups in the European Union: a consensus statement. Euro Surveill 2014;19(9):pii=20728. Article DOi: http://dx.doi. org/10.2807/1560-7917.eS2014.19.9.20728
14. Belgian tuberculosis register 2013, Fares asbl, March 2015.
15. Dheda K, Barry Ce 3rd, Maartens G. Tuberculosis. Lancet 2015 Sep 13. pii: S0140-6736(15)00151-8. doi: 10.1016/S0140-6736(15)00151-8.

16. Lin Pl, Flynn Jl. Understanding latent tuberculosis: a moving target. J Immunol 2010 Jul 1; 185(1):15-22.

17. Salgame P, Geadas C, Collins l, Jones-lopez e, ellner JJ et al. latent tuberculosis infection--Revisiting and revising concepts. Tuberculosis (edinb). 2015 Jul; 95(4):373-84.

18. Van Zwanenberg. The influence of the number of bacilli on the development of tuberculous disease in children. Am Rev Respir Dis 1960 Jul; 82: 31-44.

19. Borgdorff Mw, Sebek M, Geskus RB, Kremer K, Kalisvaart N, van Soolingen D et al. The incubation period distribution of tuberculosis estimated with a molecular epidemiological approach. Int J Epidemiol 2011 Aug; 40(4):964-70.

20. Steingart KR, Schiller I, Horne DJ, Pai M, Boehme CC, Dendukuri N. Xpert® MTB/RiF assay for pulmonary tuberculosis and rifampicin resistance in adults. Cochrane Database Syst Rev 2014 Jan 21; 1:CD009593. doi: 10.1002/14651858.CD009593.pub3.

21. Maynard-Smith l, larke N, Peters JA, lawn SD. Diagnostic accuracy of the xpert MTB/RiF assay for extrapulmonary and pulmonary tuberculosis when testing non-respiratory samples: a systematic review. BmC Infect Dis 2014 Dec 31; 14: 709. doi: 10.1186/s12879014-0709-7.

22. Automated real-time nucleic acid amplification technology for rapid and simultaneous detection of tuberculosis and rifampicin resistance: xpert MTB/RiF assay for the diagnosis of pulmonary and extrapulmonary TB in adults and children. World Health Organisation 2013.

23. Stoffels K, Allix-Béguec C, Groenen G, wanlin M, Berkvens D, Mathys V, et al. From multidrug- to extensively drug-resistant tuberculosis: upward trends as seen from a 15-year nationwide study. PloS One 2013 May 9; 8 (5): e63128. doi:10.1371/journal.pone.0063128.

24. Ma Z, Lienhardt C, Mcilleron H, Nunn AJ, Wang X. Global tuberculosis drug development pipeline: the need and the reality. Lancet 2010 Jun 12; 375 (9731):2100-9.

25. Mitchison DA. Role of individual drugs in the chemotherapy of tuberculosis. Int J Tuberc lung Dis 2000; 4(9):796-806.

26. Dorman Se, Johnson Jl, Goldberg S, Muzanye G, Padayatchi N, Bozeman l, et al. Tuberculosis Trials Consortium. Substitution of moxifloxacin for isoniazid during intensive phase treatment of pulmonary tuberculosis. Am J Respir Crit Care med 2009 Aug 1; 180(3):273-80.

27. Conde MB, Efron A, loredo C, De Souza GR, Graça NP, Cezar MC, et al. Moxifloxacin versus ethambutol in the initial treatment of tuberculosis: a double-blind, randomised, controlled phase ii trial. Lancet 2009; 373 (9670):1183-9.

28. Merle CS, Fielding K, Sow OB, Gninafon M, lo MB, Mthiyane T, et al. OFlOTUB/Gatifloxacin for Tuberculosis Project. A four-month gatifloxacin-containing regimen for treating tuberculosis. N Engl J med 2014 Oct 23; 371(17):1588-98.

29. Gillespie SH, Crook AM, McHugh TD, Mendel CM, Meredith SK, Murray SR, et al. ReMoxTB Consortium. Four-month moxifloxacin-based regimens for drug-sensitive tuberculosis. N Engl J Med 2014 Oct 23; 371(17):1577-87.

30. Jindani A, Harrison TS, Nunn AJ, Phillips PP, Churchyard GJ, Charalambous S, et al. RiFAqUiN Trial Team. Highdose rifapentine with moxifloxacin for pulmonary tuberculosis. N Engl J med 2014 Oct 23; 371(17):1599-608.

31. RIEDER H, Comment combattre la tuberculose en 2000, Ed.Respiration.. .1998

32. Diarra B. Etude des Connaissances, Attitudes et Pratiques Comportementales de la Population Générale de Bamako face à la Tuberculose. *Thèse de Méd. Bamako: Université de Bamako; 2004; 111.*

33. Podeme Kimonde N. Niveau de connaissance de la population du quartier Ngombe-kinkusa (Congo) sur les mesures préventives de la tuberculose. *Dissertation in Health Sciences. Kinshasa - Ngaliema. Université pédagogique nationale; 2009,* 49.

34. Ministry of Planning. Equête Démographique et de Santé RDC, 2014.

35. Ouédraogo M, Kouanda S, Dembélé M, Ouédraogo SM, G. Badoum, Ouédraogo G et al. Obstacles to the implementation of directly observed treatment in the city of Ouagadougou, Burkina Faso. *Int J Tuberc Lung Dis 2006; 10: 188-91.*

36. Ottmani S, Obermeyer Z, Bencheikh N, Mahjour J. Knowledge, attitudes and beliefs about tuberculosis in urban Morocco. *La Revue de Santé de la Méditerranée orientale 2000; 14: 2.*

37. Deribew A, Abebe G, Apers L, Jira C, Tesfaye M, Shifa J et al. Prejudice and misconceptions about tuberculosis and HIV in rural and urban communities in Ethiopia: a challenge for the TB/HIV control program. *Deribew et al. BMC Public Health 2010; 10:400.*

38. Christina M, Bacay-Domingo N, Lisa Ong-Lim A. A descriptive study of the knowledge, attitudes and practices on tuberculosis among treatment partners of pediatric Patients in Tarlac city. *PIDSP Journal 2009; 10:1* .

39. Zaher H, Mokhtar A, Shouman A. The meaning of tuberculosis among community members in two Egyptian governorates 1996.

40. Rita L, Ailinger. Tuberculosis knowledge among Latino-immigrants Public health and the environment. *Abstract* 85454, November 2004.

41. Portero Navio JL, Rubio Yuste M, Pasicatan M A. Socio-economic determinants of knowledge and attitudes about tuberculosis among the general population of Metro Manila, Philippines. *Int J Tuberc Lung Dis 2002; 6: 301- 6.*

42. Mushtaq MU, Shahid U, Abdullah HM, Saeed A, Omer F, Mushtaq AS et al. Urban-rural inequities in knowledge, attitudes practices regarding tuberculosis in two districts of Pakistan's Punjab province. *Mushtaq et al. International Journal for Equity in Health 2011, 10:8.*

43. Ouedraogo M, Kouanda S, Boncoungou K, Dembele M, Zoubga Za, Ouedraogo SM et al. Therapeutic itinerary of bacilliferous tuberculosis patients detected in two tuberculosis treatment centers in Burkina Faso. *Int J Tuberc Lung Dis 2006; 10: 184-7.*

APPENDIX

- Collection sheet

SOCIO-DEMOGRAPHIC PARAMETERS	
1. Age:	
2. Gender:	
3. Profession:	
4. Number of children:	
5. Religion:	*Catholic / Protestant / Revival / Others (Kimbangmste)*
6. Level of education:	*None / Primary / Secondary / University / Post-graduate*
SOCIO-ECONOMIC PARAMETERS	
7. Living conditions	
- How much do you spend on per day?	
- How much do you spend on per day?	
- How often do you eat?	
- Do you have a television?	
- Do you have a radio?	
- Do you consult the Internet from time to time? time to inform yourself?	
- Are you interested in health magazines?	
KNOWLEDGE OF TB AND THE VACCINE	
8. Do you know about TB?	*Yes / No*
9. Have you heard of TB?	*Yes / No*
10. How did you hear about this disease?	*Television /Radio / Third party / Other:*
11. What is TB?	
12. How do you get this disease?	*Contage 1d* / Contage 2d* /Other:*
13. Is this disease contagious?	*Yes / No*
14. How is it transmitted?	*By: Respiratory secretion / Sexual contact / Unprotected food / Other:*
15. How do you suspect TB in a person?	*By: a cough lasting more than 2 weeks / profound weight loss / incessant diarrhea / Other:*
16. What does a person with TB look like?	*Cough / Fever anorexia / Asthenia / Weight loss / Profuse sweating / Other:*

17. What do you do if you know someone has TB?	*We take him to the hospital / we take him to the tradipratician / we quarantine him / Other:*
18. What test is used to confirm TB?	Sputum examination / Radiology / Blood examination / Other:
19. How is it treated?	In hospital by anti-T / by antibiotic / Traditional products
20. How do you protect yourself against TB?	By vaccination / By other measures
21. Do you know about the BCG vaccine?	Yes / No
22. What is the age requirement for the TB vaccine?	
23. How and where is the vaccine administered?	
24. Are you familiar with the vaccination booklet available to mothers and did you use it when your children were born?	

FSC
www.fsc.org
MIX
Papier | Fördert gute Waldnutzung
FSC® C083411

Kolibri 360 GmbH
Ferdinand-Jühlke-Straße 7
99095 Erfurt, Deutschland
produktsicherheit@kolibri360.de

Druck:
CPI Druckdienstleistungen GmbH
im Auftrag der
Kolibri 360 GmbH
Ferdinand-Jühlke-Str. 7
99095 Erfurt